CW01636697

signs that broke me copyright © 2024 by Ciara Daly. All rights reserved.
No part of this book may be used or reproduced in any manner without written permission except in the case of reprints and the context of reviews.

I dedicate this to my sisters–
three who broke many times,
but the luckiest cards I was dealt,
to be given the chance
of having best friends for life.

table of cards

a preface for my readers

it is with a great honour that I introduce my second collection of poetry and prose, *signs that broke me*. I would love to say we're back for round two, but unfortunately, things have taken a darker turn for my second publishing venture. life isn't all fairies and rainbows, and neither is healing through spirituality. in this book, I expose the vulnerability of acknowledging my demons and what can happen when you first unearth trauma, generational curses, mental health issues and societal wounds. not surprisingly, I discovered that all the above can break a person-when you realise just how unfair the cards life has dealt you are. there wasn't much room for positivity here, but a blunt force dive into my darkness. as I battled with these demons, I turned to spiritual self-help practices to help guide me towards the light, or at least understand these difficult emotions I was feeling. hence, my inspiration for the chapters of this book became the wounded archetypes of the zodiac and the tarot cards connected to them.

each chapter represents a tarot card, zodiac sign, and an astrology house, as a general theme for the upcoming poems and traumas. tarot and astrology are therapeutic tools I refer to often, but I find tarot especially helpful on a day-to-day basis. for the most part of this book, I talk about a darkness that has lived with me for a long time (from about eight years old), generational wounds I inherited and personality disorders explained in my birth chart. this darkness has haunted me in different ways throughout my life. it has made me, broke me and awoke me, through traumatic experiences and a 'tarot like' series of events. astrology explains your psyche, karmic lessons, self-realisation and your inherent personality. in contrast, tarot will bring more insight about your life and about how the world around is affecting you here and now. tarot is attuned to your emotions, unpredictable, external influences and the fate which is out of our personal powers.

to those who haven't read my first book, it explains astrology and its basic principles. *signs to grow up* describes the planets in relation to the zodiac signs, how to read your birth chart and the basic stuff to understand about astrology, like your sun, moon and rising sign. *signs that broke me* is fewer references and more prose. this time I wanted to focus on the relatability of my poetry and life experiences, rather than spiritual concepts and explaining archetypes. this collection is about the early adult stage of my life, the realities, struggle and lost innocence, as I pick apart the experiences and relationships that broke me. like the tarot fool card who throttles themselves into the world full of hope and naivety, I found darkness awaited me once I left behind my child-like inner world. if you are looking for an introductory guide to astrology, zodiac personalities and poetic inner child experiences, read *signs to grow up*. if you are angry, lonely and want to see your traumatic experiences in words and through relatable zodiac personas, you have it coming.

during my editing process, when I questioned censorship and tactfulness, I read my favourite Rupi Kaur books, *milk and honey* and *home body*. her work reminds me that I don't have to filter my experiences, regardless of how 'trigger warning' they feel. in fact, as a trigger warning, this book is probably 200 pages worth of triggers and writing that is intended to invoke strong responses. Rupi was the first writer I encountered who put a lot of taboos out there, the first poet who wrote poetry I could understand and who put my explicit experiences in words. she has been a big inspiration for the courage and contents of this book, even structurally with lower case and times new roman font. the next question that bothered me was-is this *poetry*? many online trolls have slammed Rupi for even calling hers such. yet her 'unpoetic' words have resonated with so many women, women who need unfiltered poetry that speaks honestly. I granted myself the 'poetic' license to do the same.

an important part of understanding the benefit of these poems is that it's not true artistic poetry, but therapy. the world is full of creators, but only a few are called artists (that's not the exclusivity or level of writing I aspire to). for me, creating this was cathartic and therapeutic-when I badly needed a method of release. I think I would classify this type of writing as therapy art, to be kept in cathartic museums for mental illness. a place to be recognised, seen, or heard. still, are the words I write toxic? disturbed? do I romanticise pain? maybe so, but for me it's empowering to read about the same darkness you feel.

yet, in the process of writing, I realised I could only go so far-that stagnation is easier than growth. it is not a catharsis if you fixate on the same words, you will grow mad, worsen your condition. I knew I could not stay in this madhouse, however at home I felt.

in the end my work, while I ruminated here, was not peaceful or meditative. I felt like I had purged the madness from my mind and was left staring at pages of my own vomit. to regain perspective, I moved onto a second project, leaving this manuscript untouched for many months. reading my words can be angering and upsetting, but justifiably, sometimes people feel angry and upset. there is no easy remedy for mental illness, but therapy and forms of self-expression are a start. therapy is an honest confession, a breakdown of ugliness to show it as it is. this book I created is unmedicated and raw in its prognosis. it is the reality of a modern woman's mind, one that has suffered and one that pursues creativity in the midst of pain. if writing is an art form, mine is hard, non-fiction and I paint in blunt strokes. I know in writings to come my paintbrush and style will change, but I want to share these hardships, ones that I know others feel. women experience this and sadly, it's not spoken freely enough in order for us to normalise the pursuit of healing, enlightening and saving our broken selves.

in terms of therapy-why astrology? why tarot? because hobbies can save lives. just like other forms of psychological self-help, finding self-identity and validation can help soothe feelings of uncertainty and isolation in a healing journey. astrology is about identification-but you can also confront the dark traits in your birth chart personality. if you don't confront it within yourself, unfortunately, like all karmic principles, you'll meet this darkness in outer world experiences. this is where tarot can act as a corrective, preventative self-awareness tool. often people say trouble follows them or finds them-they are accident prone or unlucky, like pulling a tower card repeatedly. but with awareness, we can manage our weaknesses and steer the events in our life. similarly, ignorance of our shadow traits and subconscious wounds, like ignoring the death or devil card, can create destructive patterns in our lives. any healing process must start with fully, and honestly releasing the repression, guilt, anger, shame, fear and pain that we are holding in our bodies. here, through the cards and the signs, I honestly show you all of mine.

fire can be a prison
the sea offers an escape
air is ever changing
but earths are humble ground
the flames bring a passion
that the waves will swallow up
the winds are uplifting
when the earth can bury you
but too much of anything

is just enough to kill you

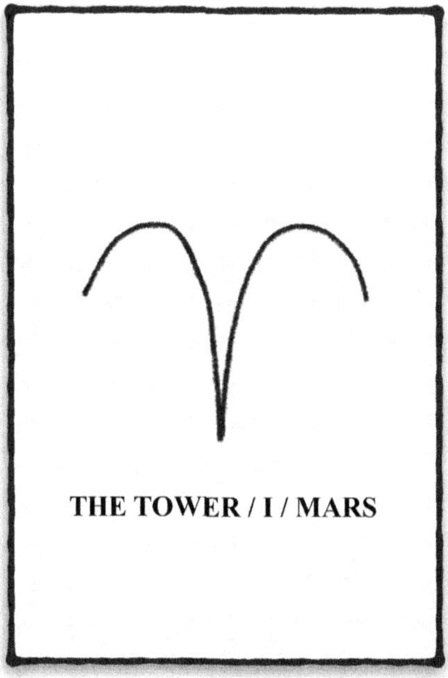

1

a deer caught in headlights
I should get a blood test
badly painted toenails
everything comes in threes
just too tough to cry
firm handshakes
biting the hand that feeds you
that's not very ladylike
flirting with another tattoo
loud chewers
one way ticket temptations
female rage when I shave
burning my toast
two wrongs don’t make a right
blunt force trauma
expecting beginner’s luck
good girl gone bad

- *aries angst*

my person and your person
just far too young
and had lives to live
the right person
at the wrong time
who broke my heart gently

before I knew what it was to cry

I always hated my red cheeks
and how they'd reveal everything
so I covered them up
with a stolen pharmacy bb cream
the price of my masculine beauty
or the first warning sign
of an anti-social personality
only for you to pass me in the hallways
an affirmation to all of the above
by putting a finger to my cheek
and hear you jeer in disgust-
look how much makeup just came off
a scarlet shame stuck to me
and a deep-rooted rage
that even when I try to hide it

I'll never be beautiful enough

heart on my sleeve
blood pooling at the cuffs
I didn’t want to make a scene
dripping all over the carpet
and stumbling to stitch myself together
did I always exude an air
that I don’t need any help
since you stayed behind the yellow tape
while my hands were tied
to be taken out in a body bag
with rug burn from where I cried

effort was a one way street
where I paved the way
and you marked your steps
before my sentiment
had enough time to dry

at night when I close my eyes
and try count sheep to get to sleep
instead of dreams
the first thing that comes to mind
someone just stabbed me
ciara got stabbed
my name repeated in bloody red lines
so when I wake up every morning
and see the same moles and birth marks
to identify a dead girl's body
I'm reminded of who I could have been
if I wasn't born karmically
the type a baptism can't clean
so the first thought that comes to mind
from the nightmares of a past life
when I meet a dead girl in the mirror
is that I shouldn't be *alive*

why do I ask myself
these hypothetical questions
that if I had to pick
between my sisters being assaulted
or myself taking it again
I would go ten times over
since the blood of battle is thicker
than the waters of womanhood
I've fought before, I'll do it again

then have her touched instead

why does post-traumatic stress
feel like main character syndrome
when I walk through my hometown
and the memories strip me
naked from the waist
and eyes from places I can't see
laugh and taunt me
the trees whisper or so it seems
I am not one of them
there is no love for you here
just demons and skeletons
that mark their wrath on my body
you could call them scars
I'll call them stretch marks
from a psychological growth
so the past no longer haunts me

suicide watch feels
like staying in bed
for weekends on end
watching the same tv show
because the taurus in me fears
for what will happen next
although the sagittarius extremist
wants to dance and run free
except she waltzes straight into threat
better off buried in a hole
since earth signs know best
how easily the thoughts in my head
can catch flame and manifest
under a drunken ram influence
who lives with no regrets

as innocent as a flower
naïve since your budding hour
so you turn blindly
in whatever direction
some sunshine is offered

there is something
so base and brutish
about an aroused man
a wild animal
you repulse me
a hound to be hunted
you fooled me once
that was a shame on you
then to be fooled twice
a dog will always be a dog
so how could I blame you?
but luck comes three times
and I'm angry after round two
a long forgotten peace sign
load the rifle

– *I'm aiming for you*

I still think about how
If I stood in trial for your murder
I'd confess to wanting to stab you
a thousand more times
just to satisfy the anger
that pierced through me like knives

to feel ashamed of myself
when I receive sympathy
I run away from things
that remind me I’m vulnerable
their love stings with poignance
but if I just let people in

maybe I wouldn’t feel so broken

signs that broke me

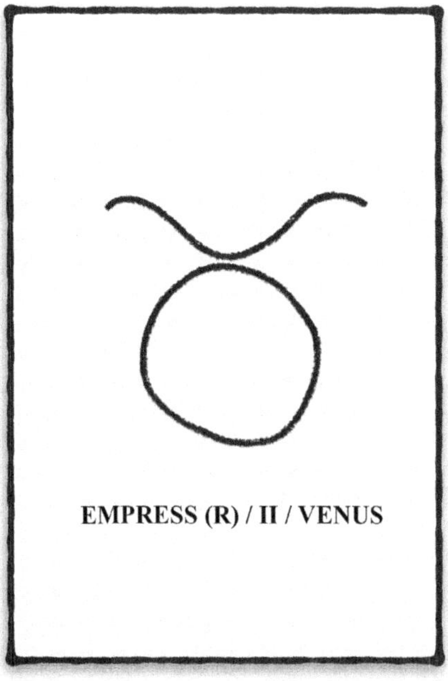

2

boys who won't commit
stuck in the forbidden forest
crying when I break a nail
finding a therapist
hopeless romantic syndrome
a teddy bear pinned to a truck
my feelings for dinner
the calm before the storm
a blocked throat chakra
have you tried exercising more?
thick with emotion
seven thing I hate about you
beauty is pain darling
an unreturned favour
pointing the finger
a bunch of overripe bananas
six feet under mentality
no more second chances

- *taurus trauma*

a childhood crime scene
the first blood stain
on my tuesday knickers
the lifelong reminder
of ruining your favourite pair
to be thrown a maxi pad
and told to hide the pain
the first sign of womanhood
was to feel ashamed
that to develop early was weak
now I forever hate
the second day of the week

you’re afraid the truth
will hurt my feelings
in all honesty
don't worry–

your *lies* already did

you might be the only asset I ever own
the little security you can give me
the type that others inherit so easily
while I used you like an office
you drove me through my favourite drive-thru
when my social paranoia got the best of me
still half bedridden in pyjamas
to get my morning coffee
and we sat and watched normal people walk
we chose peace together
so that your engine warmed my heart
with each stalled week and month
where we dropped more in value
in response to a society that times our worth
I sat and read through pages of another world
to enjoy the simplicity of the passenger seat
when I would dissociate
for days that rolled into one another
but your wheels would keep turning
and I figured if chance took my life
it would be me and you together

I was trying to figure out
how to sustain myself
on the morsels that you fed me
without feeling hungry
still I collected your crumbs
and baked a happier pie in my mind
that lead me to think the bare essentials
was enough to feel satisfied
only to realise
what I was imagining
didn't exist in real life
and when I took back everything
that was mine
I left a hollow crust behind

I am mourning a parent
who is still alive
but as I became an adult
my innocence couldn't be protected
now I see you in a different light
did age disintegrate to this
or were you always this way
I wish I could go back
to those sweet protected days
when your love was still untainted
when I still made you smile
before I was old enough to see
your mentality came with an expiry
and one day it would peak
by the use by date
in my childhood memories

emotionally uninvolved fathers
create daughters
who couldn't develop
a sense of inner security
so now we look for it in other men

I'm familiar with pain
she's the girl next door
they say regression
is another symptom to diagnose
that's why I keep speaking to her
over the wall
to see what she knows
but now, nobody plays anymore
I just want to go back
to primary school
is loss all part of my growth?

while I was stuck in the past
building bonds for the future
a place where I could ground
so you could breathe
you vanished into thin air
and I jump to answers usually
but I stumbled to realise

we just weren't meant to be

and the universe would make me pay
for being cruel in another soul
throwing my only evidence in bin bags
my favourite jacket
please god no
the devil took my body
but let me hold onto it's clothes
a false sense of protection
that time and time again proved worthless
but in my early trauma response
I got attached to physical things
when change and crisis took place

the definition of madness
is doing the same thing
again and again
and expecting things to change
is that why
when constantly defending your name
only to be disrespected again
in sickness and in health
a life cycle of hopeful disappointment
until self-preserving death do us part
since keeping our relationship alive
drove me so mad
that I broke my own heart

the strongest daughter
that walked the earth in my life
who felt everything physically
you always told me
that shaving your legs
made you feel pretty
but you never told me
when indulging in the pink tax
on overpriced razors
only to let venus touch your wrist
how did you feel?
or how young were you really
in this masculine economy
when they started to profit
off of your insecurities?

even after the pain
and all the fear that it caused me
the biggest blow
was hearing silence from the people
who saw the blood streaming down my legs
and heard me scream for help
only to turn and tell me how serious it was
to accuse someone of *rape*

you told me I was strong
but it would have been
much more comforting to know
that the weight I was carrying
was much too heavy
for such small shoulders

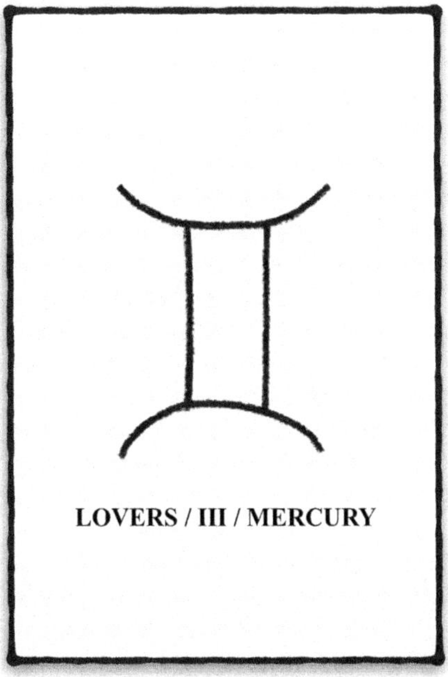

3

romantic red flags
remembering random facts
switching sides
what if I loose my sparkle?
awkward silences
thinking instead of sleeping
forgetting to feed myself
mind over matter
why are you so slow at replies
the butterfly taking effect
playing sims as an adult
not smelling the gaslighting
breathing exercises
screwing the plot of my life
the cause or the cure
please just take me seriously
a three year itch
what was I made for?

- *gemini grief*

you're not intentionally cruel
but you force my fragility
into a disclosure of hope
that never results in anything
as if you would have me bare
my wounds
for the pleasure of looking
without the intention
or power to heal it

I watched you dance into one room
and put on a show
then walk into the next one
and start playing a different role
I had a personality disorder
what was your excuse for?
thing is I think we were so very close
to really knowing each other

falling in love
with both of your sides
meant I set myself up
for unrequited polygamy
did I have '*cheat on me*'
stuck on my forehead
this whole time
I should of known this would happen
when you mix *venus* and *gemini*

I tend to find myself in dark places
once out of curiosity
but no longer as a visitor
since now they feel so familiar to me

– the shadow side of me

how young was I when I learned
to compromise with others
when there was no alternative
to being understood

I only pick at old wounds
because your avoidance
is a repetitive bandage
you will never heal this way
and your healing directly affects me
because you are the soul who made me

your interest of the moment
meant you dropped everyone else
to look at the smaller picture
and put on another mask
to pose for disposable feelings
a sign that you never pictured well
for a smile only a mother could love
I realised a sign of weakness in a man
is to attempt to wear the pants
and put on a different pair every time
so in time I could never lust
over the chameleon complacency
of erratic self-invested behaviour
that you captioned as trust
and the longer I look at the picture
the uglier you become

cure and the cause
since the people
who should be curing me
are the cause
of what's wrong with me

a soft scam
or soft cheating
where there is a full spectrum
between right and wrong
a world that we live in where
it’s so easy to be deceived
and so typical to be wronged

I am haunted with déjà vu
through everyday things
like drinking sugar-free drinks
that tricked my brain into thinking
I was getting energy
when it was actually just caffeine
another taste of trust issues
and the inevitable come down
now I only go for people
that are what it says on the tin
so I'm not artificially sweetened
into believing that you care about me

it is time to realise
that their behaviour is no longer triggering
since they will never change
they have become the *trigger*
you just have to accept it and walk away

vanity gets the best of me
and any water sign will see through
my captions that lack integrity
or any deeper meaning
because all I want is to see the lightness
of myself in this world
I couldn't handle anything less
like discovering I had a shadow trait
but would I be happier if I knew instead?

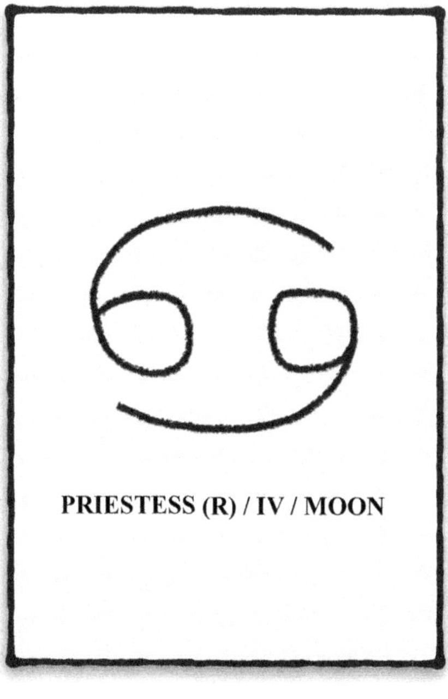

4

how to disappear
the subjectivity queen
fighting for this love
it's time to change the bedsheets
chronic period pains
I can walk myself down the aisle
voluntary house arrest
the low-fat milk for mommy
an empty first aid kit
playing sad music when I'm sad
carrying water weight
whatever love means
who taught me to hide my tummy
working on man-made time
a love like ariana and mac
I just want my own home
come back jack

- *cancer cries*

life becomes easier
once you accept
that men will disappoint you
at every stage
at any age

to all the women
and their responses
who were once little girls
that didn't know what trauma meant
but lost themselves in fantasy novels
to disappear inside their own head
the same woman who obsess
about movies, music and characters
by using their first coping mechanism
to find a way to escape

I saw you looking at her
before you were done seeing me
a sidelined torture
where out of the blue she comes
but once you know you know
that's why they call her–

the other woman

a muffled scream
a stifled sob
a leaky faucet in the shower
where no one can hear me
my morning alarm
wakes a tear-soaked pillowcase
bittersweet chocolate chips
to numb a first heartbreak
a sweet extract like vanilla
the type I never weigh
when I pour it into my cupcakes
another beautiful mistake
filled to the brim
how much more till I sink
though I still manage to rise
I'll know tomorrow morning
if everything tastes ok
and I wake to a dry pillowcase

I spent so much time
trying to be your rose
only to realise
I was playing juliette
to a worthless romeo

the effort that women make
to keep relationships afloat
planning, preparing, booking
cooking, cleaning, smiling,
teaching, caring, loving
supporting, minding, raising
excusing, condoning, forgiving
prioritising, apologising, forgetting
compensating, begging, trying
how much more must we do
for the men of our relationships
is this all that we know
growing up watching our mothers
do the the same for our fathers
or are we scared of true love
are we wary of letting go
incase loosing our control
means we have to see these sons
for who they've truly become

have you ever tried intermittent fasting
for six teenage years of school
I didn't eat from nine-to-four
and threw my sandwiches
in the sanitary pad bins
because I felt too ashamed to eat
around underdeveloped boys
in case they called me fat
and thus began the foreshadowed fling
there in the bathroom stalls
of my ten-year-affair with bulimia

did you get too carried away
in your divine masculine
that you forget to thank
the feminine that feeds you
or perhaps you never did
expecting to be cared for
and loved
but is it really egalitarian
if after the working day
she is often scheduled
for so much more
but I'm sorry
if I stopped making an effort
or put on a few pounds
how could I possible expect
with my moods and whims
to ask for gratitude or respect

please if there is a god out there
give me another chance
at feeling whole again
send another one of your angels
to fill this void
the last one left

the girl who destroyed herself
to forget about the part
you made her give up
her last words as she left
forget about me
the repercussions are haunting
since you heard her name
while you slept with me
and left memories on your pillow
so I would never forget
and carry her pain
taken from one to another
even though we weren't ready
the type that can only be carried
inside of a woman's body

I wonder could a psychic tell me
the only thing I don't know
if I’ll go down the aisle in white
before I turn forty
in a coffin or a dress

I have to be grateful
that things could be worse
yet in my trauma response
I never relearned how to enjoy sex
from the day
my autonomy was taken away
I was sentenced to a life
of never truly enjoying intimacy again
having to repeatedly remind myself
that *you are safe*
having to expose damaged places
that will never be the same
a medusa turned to stone
sometimes feeling like a duty
my *lust* was taken away that day

it was painful to watch
you try assert your self
to an unreceptive audience
of the emotionally intelligent
when I knew your heart was in the right place
but you didn't have the right words to say
and sometimes those three little words
have the power between
leaving and staying
but you were three words too late

– I love you

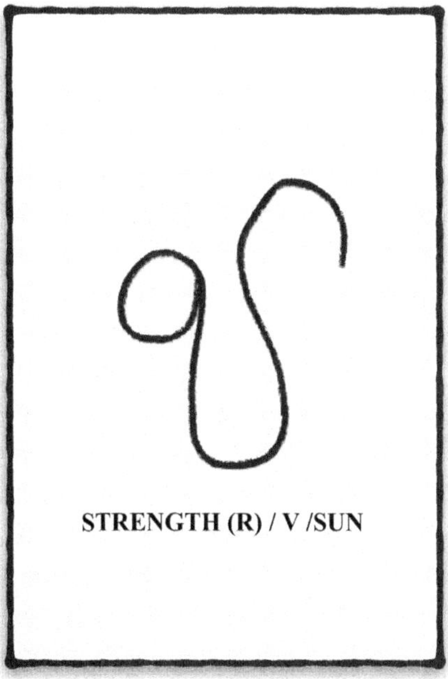
STRENGTH (R) / V /SUN

don't touch my hair
waiting for the sun to rise
a beautiful liar
high blood pressure texts
imposter syndrome
smile though your heart is aching
arrogant affirmations
almost is never enough
love bombing
throwing away the key
catcalled on the street
constructive criticism bruises
I'll take your man
hearing it disrespectfully
a volcano on standby
the cat has claws
my inner child still screams

- *leo liabilities*

there are three people in life–

the fighter
the protector
or the protected

and I'll never come third

it was very difficult to watch
a child that was beeped at
by fully grown peeping toms
a liability to the road
while she walked home
wearing her school uniform

I have way too much pride
locked up in my own castle
from a fear of pettiness
and a preconception
that it's not my duty
to reveal how I truly feel

when did you know you weren't ok?–

my sister said my smile
didn’t match my eyes

no I don’t think your crazy
except it’s just the way
and the lengths you went to prove
he had moved on
because you couldn't understand
more like accept
that he couldn't want you

so it must be someone else

I hired you into my life
without checking references
or seeing certificates
another under-qualified lie
when I tried to manage
a skill set that never existed
doing overtime to compensate
for an emotional language
of broken sentences
to fill disconnected silences
and feeling inadequate
from asking you to apply yourself
to the bare minimum

do we need to break up
so I can find my self-worth
since I hated myself so much
is that why I put off leaving
to prove that I was worthy enough
the queen of avoidance
and paranoia my regal advisor
where we couldn't come down to earth
to realise
your love was not enough

you told me I'd be more attractive
a few kilograms lighter
a week before my graduation date
so I hated all the pictures
half a stone too heavy
then you gifted the extra weight
wrapped inside a golden necklace
could I forget what you said?
in a warped love language
where gift giving
could make everything ok?

then my first college holiday
I weighed less than a twelve-year-old
so scared of a bikini
that I left my dinner in a toilet
it took a boy twice my height
to put me on his shoulders
only to slap at my leg
and say that I was getting too heavy
god, if only then
atop my wounded throne
or locked inside the bathroom stall
could I have seen the irony

is there anything more viscous
than the insults you throw
at a younger sister
who has stolen your clothes
probably because boys from my school
watched a film about mark zuckerberg
and compared the girls in class
with a spreadsheet on microsoft word
happy that I marked higher than worst
did I become conditioned to think
that bodies are just bodies
and to state the obvious
from one size to the next
without realising the feelings connected
to seams, lines and shapes

‘you were hungry’
‘you enjoyed that’
‘didn’t you just eat?’
‘I could never eat all that’
‘you're still hungry?’

passing comments at dinner like table salt
you carved away at my pride
and you wondered why we started eating alone
or tiptoed to get a snack
why was a basic human requirement
served as something so shameful to us?

why did you have to distort your brain
and numb your reality
to show me warmth and affection?

– *a love language in disconnection*

was I naïve as a puppy
to fall for someone else's show?
the type I orchestrate
a role I played many times before
in my greed, in my lust
and all my self-centred glow
the cat should have known
that everything that glitters
isn't always gold

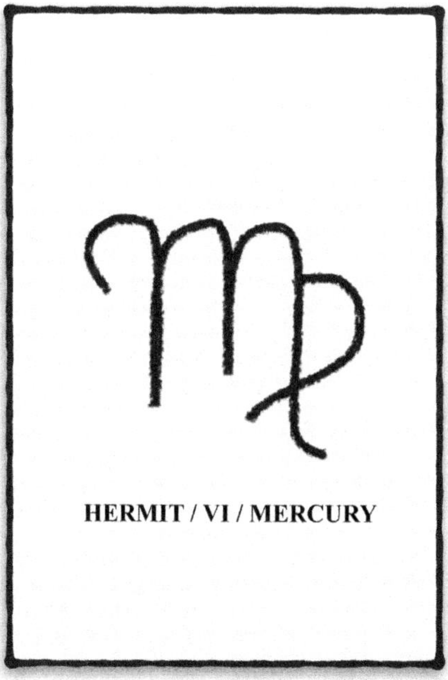

6

jumping to conclusions
the smell of bleach
when did I last have a dream
karmic debt nineteen
acting your wage
checking yours before mine
monica from friends
a smooth criminal
speaking at me not to me
paralysis from analysis
how to pamper practically
I can feel it in my gut
jeans and a nice top
right words in the wrong tone
picking your poison
asking for help
emotionally unavailable men

- *virgo vices*

7

messy personal spaces
since they say your private time
is a reflection of your inner mind
so when my mental health starts to give
and my room becomes a mess again
I dress to look like
I-have-everything-under-control

so that no one will ever know

the truth about having
an adult boyfriend
in my childhood bedroom
is that he will never know
the little girl who lived here
that suffered in silence
for sleepless nights spent crying
within four pink painted walls
the same place where
a girl became a teenager
then that teenager nearly grew up
but had to become a child once more
in order to do so
is it sad because he will never know
how much I cried
how much I escaped
how many times I felt safe
felt trapped
felt ashamed
as the little girl I was before
in this childhood bedroom
with peeling paint from years ago

I found myself with the same men
who reacted with no emotion
when I was hurt or broken
and had nothing to give
other than anger and motivation
to put emotion into action
and do the right things for me
but if you could of stopped
and opened your soft side
that you managed so strictly
I would have felt safer
then all your repressive tendencies

– *daddy issues*

I am not sure he understands
that people need emotional intimacy
but I know he can feel it
is that supposed to be enough for me?

watching the person who fought
for everyone else but themselves
start to give up in the very small ways
that they put up their own fight
makes me wonder
which one of us goes first

when my ptsd started kicking
I ground it down
and mixed it with mismatched mechanisms
then condensed it into a rolling paper
to light it like a cigarette
and stress smoked till I stopped dreaming
of things I wanted to forget
to deal with those disorderly feelings

I pick boys who need me
so they will never leave me

I know we have healed
the inner child
but since we can never leave her
in our reverse learning
why did you teach us
that it was ok
to accept men
who can’t express themselves
we understand them too much
recognise them so much
love them so much
because they raised us
with so little emotion
yet we still felt loved

how can I heal
or show the doctor where it hurts
because I still feel the bruises
black and blue insides
from where you touched me
are these my best years
or will I only live through the worst
why is happiness so hard
but so effortless to those
who have nothing to overcome
or who can watch their wounds heal
without the internal confession
of where they came from

I have been calling
for years at a time
on disconnected phone lines

you never explained why

for the fathers
that body shamed our mothers
was that another method
of your off-hand parenting
to prepare us
for the harsh reality
of how another son
would treat us in the real world

– *objects*

I will do anything
to show that I love you
except say it

you say you want a slice of this pie
I could say it was a piece of cake
but that would be a lie
since if I showed you the ingredient list

you would loose your appetite

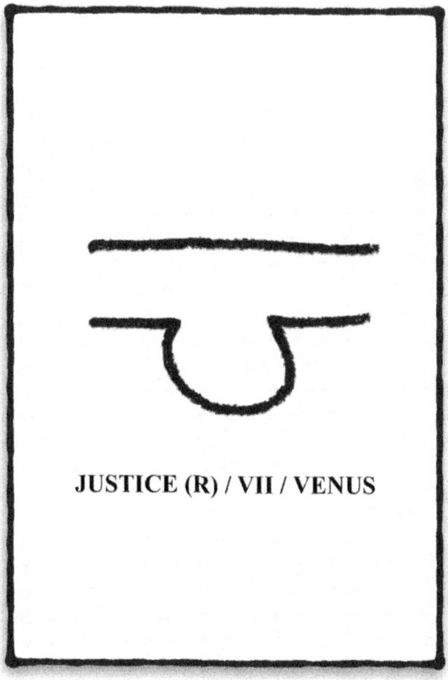

8

the honeymoon phase
pros and cons list
I think I caught a cold again
balancing the bathroom scales
a car window as a mirror
karmic debt sixteen
more than meets the eye
luxuries instead of groceries
flirting by accident
passive aggressive tendencies
an overactive heart chakra
loneliness is my biggest fear
taking screenshots of everything
rose-tinted glasses
seeking warmth in other people
subtle shapeshifter
saying yes instead of no

- *libra lies*

9

that popping tag satisfaction
that's why I bought lots of clothes
window shopping alone
wearing all my diamonds
as my material best friend
where we plan outfits in my head
from the latest fashion week model
until all the same feelings
like a change in the seasons
return with an empty basket
when they go out of trend

– *retail therapy*

one of my most distinct childhood memories
was stepping on the bathroom scales
in my granny's house, on my mother's side
and running around the perimeter of the house
once, twice and finally ten times
then stepping back on
until I saw the number change
I hadn't reached my eighth birthday
but knew that being thin over fat
meant you were admired superiorly
in a place where I was supposed to feel safe

girls will be bitches
and boys will always be boys
but you will meet girls
yet they will not be girl’s girls
taught without having to talk
by their masculine mothers
and you'll learn what that means
when you’re all grown up

I traced the fine lines
of an adult colouring book
between peace and justice
where either way all that mattered
was that I kept my colours inside

– *self-control*

I could be a celebrity
but only if you accept me
the words I see when I read her mind
the girl who so often has to redefine
her idea of beautiful
and leaves little to the imagination
behind perfectly posed pictures
but little do we know
every single comment and assumption
to her matters the most

I was so angry
that I couldn't get the justice I deserved
and I became ruthless
to every subsequent slight or disrespect
my wounded soul thought it heard

how many more times
must I endure the pain
of watching my daughters
walk through my door
with tear-stained cheeks
souvenirs from the sons
you failed to make men

– *girl dads*

it's sick that ignorant friends
avenge your imaginary innocence
and torment me
in bouts of sleep paralysis dreams
this is the educated reality
of how post-traumatic stress
can unassumingly manifest
through the blind loyalty
and dirty looks
of society's sexist best friend

life isn't fair
even when we made it more
by telling girls they could do
everything that boys are raised up for
life really isn't fair
how boys never stop being mothered
since when they grow up
girlfriends replace their mother's role
but life really wasn't fair
when little girls with brothers
had been raising themselves
many years before
how can I every find fairness
in a world where I'm set up
to accept and receive so much less
unless I submit to a feminineness
and support the men instead

– *feminine energy*

you told me to stop believing
everything I read
but everything I read was true
so maybe you wanted to hide
the truth about me and you

when a police officer told me
I had insufficient evidence
I felt like ripping my heart out
on his interrogation table
to have it tagged and sealed
with the labels they gave my words
placed inside an evidence bag
and sent away for testing
just to find a way
to prove that you broke me

a picture without a frame
since even if we tried
it would shatter into pieces
and a memory in tatters
seems better kept
than to hang seven years back luck
wearing our sundays best
just to smile through the cracks
a reflection
that there is nothing of us left
it takes the toughest child to realise
that appearances are lies
and behind closed doors
hides the unhappiest memories

– *broken families*

if I just take the medications
and submit to society's idea of balance
will I be happier
from settling for so little
I sell my body and mind for pennies
because I think I'm worth nothing
I would put my life on the sale rack
my skills and talents
my energy and time
my opinion and counsel
at a reduced rate
even though in the mania of fashion week
I feel like hot shit
but then off-season comes
and I sink to the bottom of the pile
worn and washed out hundreds of times
ready to take the first buyer
dump me in a bag
my seams and folds caving in
why do I take trends to the extreme

– I just want to find peace

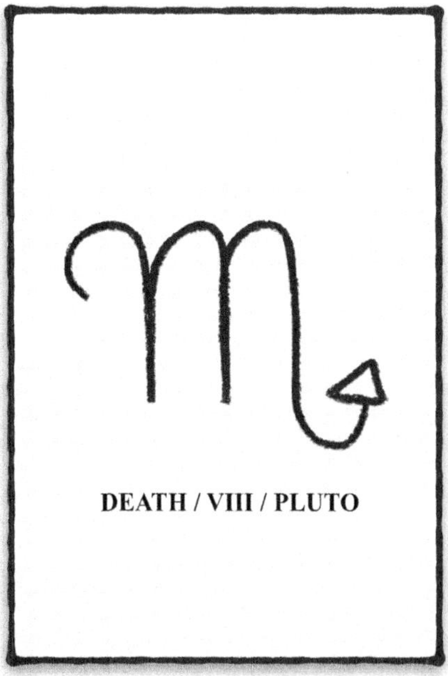

10

hot and cold
did my intensity scare you
mourning my past self
seven minutes in heaven
living in my head rent free
I need louder earphones
coffee that burns my tongue
toxic femininity
nobody takes me softly
transformation expiry dates
hour long showers
playing with fire
the nail in my coffin
a sadistic kiss from pluto
it comes in waves and storms
taking revenge as therapy
the wrong hole

- *scorpio scars*

your temperament was offensive
still you adored any attention
and god were you a bore
even when there was nothing there
knowing I hated letting go
paired with an attention whore
it's like you were too selfish to say

I don't like you anymore

my scorpio best friends
who weren't there for me in the end
rhetorically, was pain and suffering
all just part of your DNA
that dying and rebirthing yourself
was something so inherent
to not feel empathy when I cried
or claimed I wanted to die

had the wounded scorpio in you
become so accustomed
to a life decked with darkness
and inflicted with pain
to live comfortable with destruction
you were raised on pain and suffering
so when it came to another's upset
you had nothing left to give

I always said I wouldn't follow
or misrepresent others I've met
with the stereotypes given to zodiacs
but your scars I can't forget
since it seems that every water sign
suffering between these dates
turn to stabbing me in the back
as their parting goodbye

you don't trust the world
because you don't trust yourself

what ever parts I had to match yours
they never stood a chance
and were outnumbered
by your duplicating side
like a virus that spread and multiplied
then one day you shrivelled up
and left me from the inside
taking the life and soul
from my jaded and stripped corpse
to move onto your next host

erotic dreams
a vessel for your anger
did it feel good?
wear that dress it fits you well
whatever to make you want me
you filled me with that fantasy
fake as it was
the feelings were real
a moment on the lips
since you were made a villain
from a lifetime of trauma tips
a happy ever after gone wrong
yet, I always pick toxic boys
so I don't feel alone

hot but then cold
when I loose all feeling
no one asks where my outfit is from
because I guard all my secrets
in a house of underlying meaning
and hoard pretty skeletons in a closet
that's why I'm prone to scheming
and a knock on the eighth door
for the day I answer my best friend
with a birth chart in scorpio
if you want to know who I am
that's one secret I'll never tell

– xoxo

if you were my best friend
why did you stick
your fingers down my throat
to make me get ready quicker
and why did you see
but never mention
that I was fading into a shadow

– *toxic femininity*

murder she wrote
and she wrote with every last breath
with every bone in her body
and from flesh to ink
came blood splattered pages
revealing all her murderous memories
to find unsolved truths
where she dug up old bodies
and asked them why they did it
it was a conviction in manslaughter
that she wrote every day
because that's what trauma taught her
that evidence
no matter the form
will always get the final say

– murder on my mind

is it for an older sister to feel
like I am responsible
for the well-being of my sister
who takes my every word
and opinion as hers
the same imitation
is the highest form of flattery
but I can't help to feel disgusted
when she starts to take after me
how can I ever make up
for the second-hand disaster
of letting her watch me starve myself
and tell myself I'm not pretty
to show a body is to be altered
I'm sorry that I influenced you
to misinterpret the concept of beauty
or underestimate the power of femininity
but if I spend the rest of my life
pretending to be everything
I should have taught you to be
maybe there's still a chance for one of us
in imitated behaviour
and you'll be twice the woman for me

the revelation of shame and disgust
when you delete
those half-naked pictures of yourself
and realise
why you posted them in the first place

– *sex sells*

the patterns in every family
the darkest hue
of unspoken characteristics
that paints a few
in different brush strokes
thinking in a different tone
the inevitable traits that come
from being born a scorpio

to break is not always a bad thing
I did it so many times to know how
to destroy yourself
but in the breaking process
free yourself from hard exteriors
and shed layers of cold, cracked skin
to be at one with your vulnerability
so warmth and divine energy
can seep into the bloodstream
we must abolish the fear
of breaking
and misinterpreting
a weakness as a loss
since if you are broken there is hope
you've already seen the worst
and have strength to gain
it takes the powerful to know
that now you can start again

– *breaking*

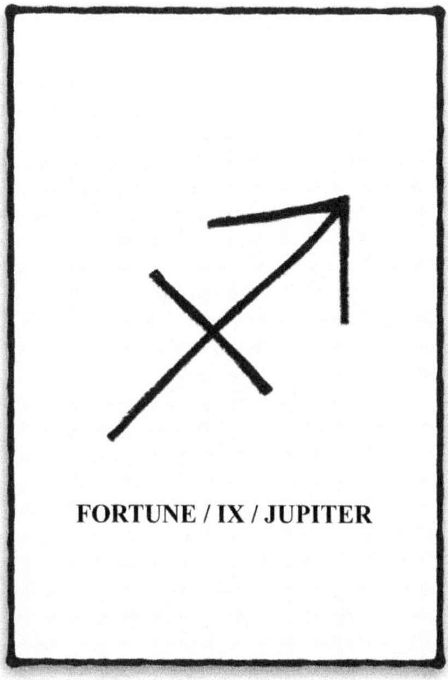

11

hook-up culture
befriending my shadow self
cutting people off again
karma is my boyfriend
food stains on a lunchbox
the last to leave the party
breaking boundaries
transferring money from savings
karmic debt fourteen
social media reels
did I just break the law
a pirate in a princess world
why can’t I love my thighs
over-exaggerating tendencies
falling from cloud nine
crimes of passion
can you please forgive me

- *sagittarius sadness*

12

a power house of astrology
where she always found the energy
for days of work, kids and activities
but to feed her fire with water
made room for psychological problems
ignored, only to be followed
by the children who took after her
that's how a little girl becomes–

her mother's daughter

I am supposed to be
keeping you at arms length
but I keep bending my elbows

– *boundaries*

your mother did it before you
to harbour the envy and lust
and compare yourself negatively
to your prettier sisters
and wear it round your neck like a chain
unearthed feelings and insecurity
propelled by vanity and beauty
your own walk of shame
to rely on the doting of other men
until you come to terms with the truth
and the resentment you had
for the divine feminine
in your inherited sister wounds

I got assaulted in a pair of skinny jeans
I bought when I was fourteen
surely I had learned my lesson then
only to be reprimanded
in my favourite tracksuit pants
I still can’t talk about the time in pyjamas
or how I couldn't feel comfortable
undressing my body for years after

don’t ever believe false realities
or let resiliency worn as blind optimism
trick you into thinking your body is safe
in anything from boys or men
since we’re told little boys were mean
because they fancy us
but they grow up to tug at skirts
of girls twenty years younger than them

if this is the only way
I can hold my perpetrators accountable
then let them burn
through books, words and written prose
the truth can't hide
and I tell myself I can heal my story
by slut-shaming your lies

– taking back what's mine

growing up around women
who always seemed to bring it back
to what she was wearing
how her hair looked
isn’t she glowing?
she lost weight but doesn’t she look great?
how well the outfit wore her
until I became the girl
who struggled to style her hair
or brush her teeth properly
not to mind painting her face in the morning
I know I should feel bad for distancing myself
from my family tree
but it had gotten exhausting
waking up to a vain mother’s day
of being another pretty leaf
and a girl I was never supposed to be

‘I’m dangerous after a drink’
‘I’m such an alcoholic’
‘I ruined my life last night’

to put myself in situations
that I count my blessings I didn’t die
I abused my family at a funeral
over too many glasses of wine
I was assaulted on my sister’s birthday
trying to get a drunk taxi home

we are not the same

the thoughts that keeps me up at night
the type a mortal human has no control over
if I hadn't been hurt
would I still have developed these disorders?

in my villain era
for retaliating to the harassment
of being singled out by a superior man
with two daughters of his own
in a fully rostered workplace
just because he can

why none of those boys
could get aroused for me
it's like something
was physically screaming
please you're not ready
even though my mind
was forcing my body

I made myself sick
because I felt physically *full*
of my emotion, trauma, memories
but when I overate to numb it
the pressure became too much
I had to feel *empty*
to purge myself of the excesses
and stress inside my body

– *bulimic tendencies*

no one is out to get me
more than myself
since it would be much easier
to find the right help
if I hadn't spent years
in a self-destructive cycle
of mania convincing myself
that I am cured
that this time I'm better
to downplay and dismiss
and tell everyone I'm healed
so when depression hits
I start all over again
will it be weeks or months
having to redefine myself
and accept getting help
before I self-destruct again

– *my own worst enemy*

signs that broke me

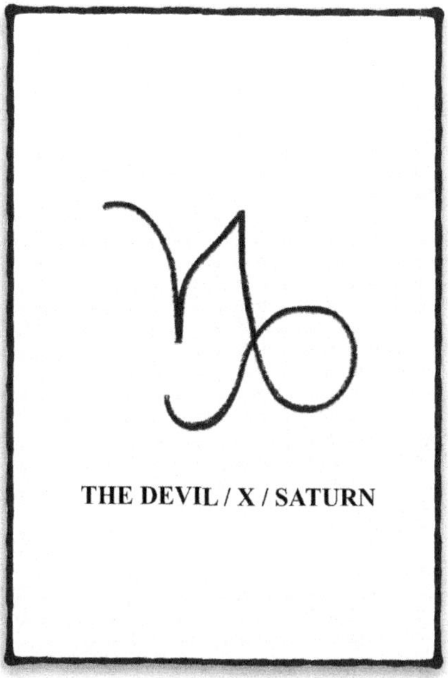

13

cathartic creativity
being told you try too hard
dancing with the devil
seasonal depression in summer
working to fill the void
therapy didn't work for me
how much is an exorcism?
an awkward dancer
finding abbreviations cringey
being scapegoated
time is my enemy
telling myself I hate kids
statistically speaking
offended by 'no offence'
a place in this world for me
hating group projects
karmic difficulties

- *capricorn crimes*

the arrested development
of a traumatised child
who can’t celebrate the same
at the milestones of her birthday
constantly playing catch up
when we are learning autonomy
that others did growing up
because in the years
when everyone was dreaming
then showing up in the world
I was tensed tight in fear
fighting off demons
that shouldn't have ever lived here
life is harder for those
who must learn availability
that others did at ten-years-old
a childhood that was incomplete
I’m only beginning to understand
in the start of my twenties
whilst I compete in a world
of adults with more experience
in understanding their feelings

the last time I was this size
I was escaping down a toilet bowl
tell me why anytime I'm suffering
some way or another
my body starts to waste away
maybe for my emphasis in physicalities
I feel I must be small
to show that I am struggling
the anxiety eats away at my mind
and I naw at my existence
to take up the least amount of space
so I deserve to be alive

why are you so bitter?

because society has conditioned us
to shave our bodies clean
and be as small as we can be
so we are attractive to men
is beauty the same as innocence
which makes us look like children?

my love language
is organisation
so just this once
can I not be the one
to *plan everything*

I can't find a sense of home
in my nuclear family
a place we always felt uncomfortable
when it came down to just five
no wonder we disintegrated
when push came to shove
why we always leaned on other families
to show what home should mean to us
is this why my older sister
is traumatised to come home
disconnected from karmic parents
a place that feels anything but her own
or why sometimes I feel most safe
most nostalgic
when leaning on the shoulder
of the youngest daughter
and watching her still grow
because even as an earth sign
I see a place in her air that came after
that is safe and full of hope

all the times my family
have asked me to produce
the real me
the girl they knew as a child
but if only they knew
that she is dead and buried so deep
so that this adult could survive
and anytime I try to reproduce her–

all she can do is cry

it will be at the gates of hell
where I barter with the devil
about whether another deed of karma
will save me if I wait in turn
because I don't see
the benefit of doing good
if I don't get anything in return

if you slice down my trunk
and let my insides spill out
all you will find is donkey years
embedded in each root
of blood, sweat and fears
and a rotten-racing-heart
pumping two rates to fast
so I'll probably have cardiac disease
in the years of my later life
having lived the symbolic irony of a noose
tied to the broken branch of a birch tree
since even if I tried
my psychological dead weight
would probably be too heavy to hang free
just my luck
to survive another breath
and suffocate a stunted biological growth
in thick-tree-trunk capillaries
to think will it be worth it
when I reincarnate in the next life
but just to be ritually safe
scatter me safely
far from the the tree I came from
so my veins escape their rotten roots
the ghosts that haunt these hollow rooms
let no one from my past find me
and all the karma of this life
I have unwilling atoned for in sacrifice
no, I will grow free and please let me be
with birds chirping in my ears
in an evergreen afterlife
I will be far away
from this withering birch tree

when my my pen starts drying up
and the stagnate depression sinks in again
to tell me I'm only worth existence
if I keep writing, working, achieving
to be human is to be earning
but it's hurting my head like static
and every empty word of dissociation
only hurts me more
but when will I feel the success
when will I be enough to deserve a break
when will everything fall into place
when will I honour my mental health
my knees are about to give in
and with the waning crescent coming
shadows of a capricorn moon
with aches in my back through the twilight
I figure I'm about to cave in

– *the goat in me*

it seems a woman has
two choices in life
capitalism or patriarchy
and either one you pick
never feels right

I never felt relief in seeing a doctor
even though so articulate
I only ever felt understood
by how many notes she took down

therapy felt like a monopoly game
that I was cheated at for property
for all the pain and suffering
they offer healthcare in loansharking

free parking for making you cry
and question where you went wrong
then roll the dice on a medication leaflet
only to move two steps back in life

to get a psychological diagnosis
felt like a get out of jail free
where you miss a round in the game
just for being mentally ill

in my life path
the end always justified the means
and that's how I came to accept
all the bad things that happened to me
but the saddest part of all
is that I witness the same mentality
in a younger capricorn girl
who accepted at ten-years-old
she didn't deserve
the happiness and praise other's get
because she was darker than them

did my own sun-sign ruin me
the stone-cold cardinal
with the need to wrangle
as much as she can
out of everyone and everything
to use and abuse the system
don't hate the player, hate the game
but I hold my cards too tight
and expect it to be fair play

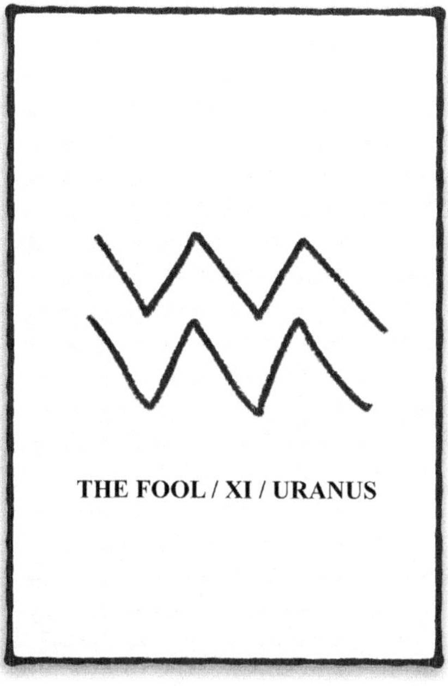

14

existential dread
overflowing laundry piles
I can’t understand my mind
barely baring
snacking my days away
picking mommy’s boys
holding everything inside
an individuality crisis
the wrong bra size
a new trend every month
mistaking charm for chivalry
a moment on the lips
I can see it in your eyes
'we're all on a spectrum'
a boner on the bus
overwatering humans
my period is late again

- *aquarius agony*

they call me the the water bearer
but sometimes I'm barely bearing
or what I meant to say
barely breathing
in a life that seems so desperate for meaning
since I sometimes can't tell the difference
between existing and feeling
and whether I exhale enough
to put so much weight into breathing
am I supposed to inhale all this air
since all I ever do is share
and I usually feel there is never enough
left over for me

I'm fine really–

I'm just an adult
still picking up the last shards
of being my family's glass child
and dealing with
the pathetic weakness
of being told you are too kind

I was lost
and looked for guidance in you
yet you threw out random life rules
to match your needs
whenever it suited you
and I had to relearn right from wrong
no wonder I was so confused

– *narcissistic abuse*

you cut my wings
then shamed me
for not being able to *fly*

your girlfriend
is not your mother
she is not your therapist
your conservator
maybe because your mother
never saw the bad in you
always forgave the unforgivable
and passed you onto me
without fully realising
the monster she conceived

– mothers and sons

I'm on top of things
until it comes to laundry day
and my basket seems empty
from shrinking my problems
as if they weren't there
even though half way through the week
I have nothing left to wear
from the endless piles
of over-worn grey matter
that infiltrate my head
but I tell my shrink things aren't so bad
wearing my cleanest sweater
I'm on top of things really
feeling my big toe poke through a hole
a few stitches to make it better
I need to colour-catch again she says
mental organisation
for when I don't have the time again
to put my problems away
I have to keep ahead of myself
to separate darks from lights
since I keep spoiling my whites
with ominous black socks
that hide between the sheets
to remind me that my innocence
is tainted by stains underneath

nobody has more staying power
more love to give
more time to sacrifice
and more sins to forgive
that a woman
who is afraid to be alone
in a society who told her so

growing up is realising
that all the bad boys
were actually mentally ill
and that all the mysterious men
were actually predatory
who prey on younger women
like animals in a jungle
attracted to the vulnerable

– sick fucks

I used to always warn
the women I know that date men
sisters, mothers, cousins and friends
that men have the mentality
of three years younger than them
even younger when it comes
to their sexual preferences
and their offences it seems
since I read in my dad's newspaper
years after the offence
that half of sexual assault victims
are under the age of eighteen

when you said
I was carrying extra weight
it took me a few years to accept
that I was heavy
with psychological pain

I'm sorry that they made you think
it was normal to cry
when taking your clothes off
since you never seemed to notice
when it brought me to tears
I knew pain travels through people
so I held tight
because this world has been evil

and hurt people *hurt* people

at first I was felt sad
for how you took
advantage of my body
but then I grieved
for how you violated
the vulnerability
of my mind

– I want my innocence back

there's the oldest sister
a beauty sent from venus
to grace the earth with her gifts
there's the youngest sister
who carries the weight of family ties
a cage is all the home bird knows
we could set her free
but where on earth would she go?
back to a cinnamon scented candle lit
that sits all alone
on a front-facing window
watching us run with the wind
while she puts out the cigarette smoke
nobody buys her flowers
but she always makes do
too busy trimming hedges
to stop and smell the roses
that the elder knows so well to grow
but the other as tough as nails
prickly like a torn
ripping through her pretty white dress
she'll take the time to cry
once she finishes mopping up their tears
to keep up with her strains
but lost in the unconscious world
she whispers to the air–

I'll fly away one of these days
(but where on earth will i go?)

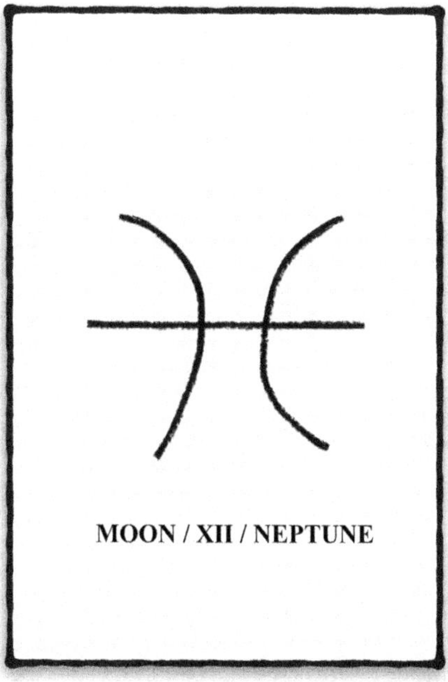
MOON / XII / NEPTUNE

keyboard warrior
maladaptive daydreaming
why do I get high off pain
the spirit in a nightcap
sorry I'm being sentimental again
karmic debt thirteen
smoking to feel like breathing
phoebe from friends
pain is the best paintbrush
self-defeatist before I start
googling a lobotomy
a justin bieber breakdown
psychologically catfished
alone in a room full of people
connection through rejection
am I a hypochondriac?
the wrong end of the rainbow

- *pisces pains*

there's nothing more melancholy
then catching the passing scent
of a woman's perfume
who used to care for you
now the trace of a stranger's waft
is all that you have left
I feel imposed to follow
and ask the name of her scent
I call it a passing melancholy
because it's all I can seem to smell

since you can't defend yourself
you defend everyone else
but you taught me
how to let others hurt me
and fail to stand up for myself
I had to relearn my self-assertion
years after the hurting
no wonder
our communication channel is broken

– passive parents

even if I amount to absolutely nothing
I have prepared myself for that
at least I've found somewhere to dream
even if I amount to absolutely nothing
I can be someone in my dreams

– what my low self-esteem tells me

for the struggling artists
who clean houses
that they will never own
for the struggling writers
who mind children
they will never have
we chose this life
self-destructive academics
that could use both sides
of the human brain
we know too much
feel too much
ignorance would be bliss
is that why the IQ of geniuses
end up smoking weed
to forget about things
or is it that the left side of life
of conformity and class
would have driven us insane

I picked broken boys
and while trying to fix them
they ended up breaking
the healer complex in me
I have to take responsibility
to make a difference in this life
but it's always the wrong kind
since I never feel good enough
when broken inside

medication leaflets
a pawn in the system
side effects worse than symptoms
my afflicted zodiac best friend
who never talked about her feelings
so I felt crazy for having them
by a wing woman who didn't fly

you always drank me under the table
already delirious on pain
and puked your heart out
then smiled like it was never there
while we suffered in silence
a clinical response to smoking
so I held my tongue to make you stay

now I wonder what happened
to make you appear so soulless
what was going on inside
a nurse with no sympathy
I checked out of an antisocial hospital
a taste of your own medicine

to act like you were never there

I shouldn't of had to kiss you
so you would leave me alone
I shouldn't of had to pretend to like you
to make you calm down
I shouldn't of had to fake it
so that it would all be over sooner
I shouldn't of had to stay quiet
to make your life easier
I shouldn't of had to live with this pain
so you could stay ignorant
I shouldn't of had to do all of the above
to be accepted by society

– to the boys who hurt me

is it my default setting
or maybe my trauma response
that every time I enter a room
I always evaluate
the fastest way to get out

I don't think it affected me that much–

*I had to close my eyes when I
washed myself for five years*

even in my safe place i couldn't *escape*

how to move out of my comfort zone
when holding back
stepping down
agreeing over arguing
avoiding stepping stones
internalising my thoughts
rationalising my dreams
all started to feel like home
just a big fish in a small bowl
who can't remember
that the wrong environment
can destroy my self-worth

I am haunted by a past
that I can never go back to
a suitcase packed tight
full of what if's
lost somewhere in transit
I cannot change
the memories misplaced
so I live with empty years
talking to imaginary friends
and reminisce
on invisible souvenirs

I'll ride this out alone
not that I would rather
but I have to
then try to confide in someone
who does not understand
the same way I feel more alone
crying myself to sleep
while lying next to someone

my heart gets broken
almost everyday
from the emotions I carry
in twelve different ways

– *pisces pains*

the author

ciara is an irish writer and an avid book-lover. in her darkest hour, she chose to write about her life experiences and all things that are close to her heart. after many breakdowns, a psychological diagnosis, and a significant amount of self-analysis and spirituality, ciara began the heavy work of confronting her trauma, shadow traits, destructive habits, and generational wounds. she put her pain to paper, so in time, when the dark dog days are over, she will never forget how far she came.

ironically, she feels safe in winter and loves the frosty weather. her favourite time of the year makes sense, it feels safe and familiar. from the moment pluto entered her sign in 2008, she experienced crises in every sense of the way. growing up in ireland in the early 2000s, meant societal expectations rarely aligned with ciara's true needs. most of her youth to early adult years were spent ignoring, deflecting and carrying a nagging, internalised feeling that something wasn't right. her spectrum of issues became all-consuming.

as a result of many failed academic pursuits, friendships and traumatic incidents, ciara realised to truly learn a valuable life lesson she had to first study herself. in a world that asks us to serve the whole first and the self second, ciara selfishly prioritised her final breakdown. sometimes we must lose everything and redefine our sense of security. sometimes being in a fragile, unknown state makes way for change and growth. despite these challenges in life, ciara wants to believe there is someone looking down on her.

after working closely with kids in recent years, ciara surprisingly loves them-but worries if she'll ever have her own. her cholesterol is often high, a recipe of both genetic disposition and too many sweet treats with her coffee. ciara chronically speaks before she thinks, but now surrounds herself with people where she can do just that. sometimes she is too materialistic and competitive, but she is working on that. she underestimates herself in abilities, worth and strength. at her worst, she envy's others for their seemingly comparatively pain-free minds and lives (she's working on that too). ciara is all or nothing, for better or for worst.

years of silence, lies and an inability to express herself has inspired ciara to find ways to help others. despite broken states, she has always bounced back with unwavering resiliency, but often too fast, too soon. an understanding that you must play the game motivates her-to play the cards you are dealt with. despite an inherent hair trigger temper (with fine hair to begin with), after writing this ciara found peace and gratitude that she is still alive to tell her stories. in the process of healing her traumas, she reflects on this book, hoping that it speaks to others who need her words.
yours truly–

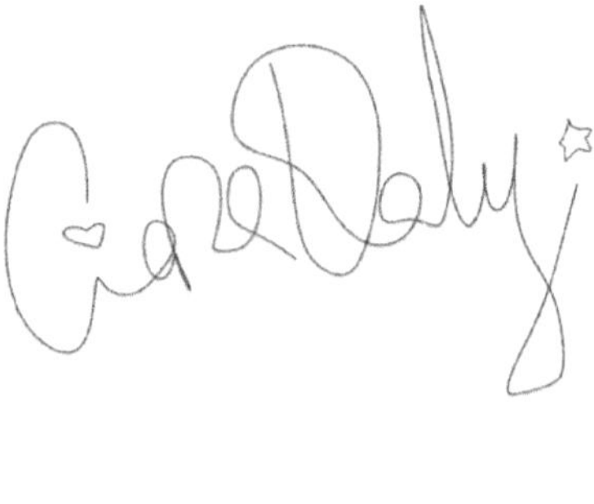

spiritual references:

[1] (i) in the tarot deck, the tower card represents sudden, unexpected changes or drastic disruptions/disasters in life. often considered a challenging card of crisis and chaos, this card can signify that sometimes we need these harsh breakdowns in order to force necessary changes or to see opportunities in life.
(ii) the first house is an area of astrology which represents our physical appearance, first impressions, self-identity, temperament, basic personality, leadership qualities and attitude towards life. this is our rising sign. anything that happens in the first house has a direct influence on our life.
(iii) mars in astrology is the planet of passion, courage, action, initiative, aggression, instincts, and our masculine energy.

[2] (i) in the tarot deck, the empress (reversed) represents the wounded archetype of mother nature, who feels out of touch with her earthly cycles, instincts and sensuality. this card also reminds us of the power of nature, how powerful its forces can be, elemental moods that can uproot our stability and security through storms, tsunamis and earthquakes.
(ii) the second house is an area of astrology which represents our concept of value, self-esteem, physical senses, materialism, possession and personal finances. our relationship with the second house can directly affect our sense of inner and outer security and our self-worth.
(iii) venus in astrology is the planet of pleasure, love, relationships, values, beauty, affection, and our feminine energy.

[3] (i) in the tarot deck, the lovers card is one of duality and represents the challenges, choices, conflicts, compromises, communication and commitment involved in romantic relationships. this card prompts us to question the consequences of love, but also take responsibility for our choices-to decide who is worthy of our love and companionship.
(ii) the third house is an area of astrology which represents social interaction, friendships, language, learning, networking, community and our early education. this house shows how we integrate socially and how we communicate or learn through our experiences with others.
(iii) mercury in astrology is the planet of communication, intelligence, skills, analysis, thought processes and logic.

[4] (i) in the tarot deck, the high priestess (reversed) represents being so immersed in the inner world and shadow self that we have become out of touch with reality. this card can suggest we are struggling to understand our feelings and must learn how to work with our dark traits so we can heal and find our higher purpose and spiritual self.
(ii) the fourth house is an area of astrology which represents domestic life, roots, ancestral patterns, caregiving, security, and the influence of your parents, especially your mother. it is a place of nostalgia and early childhood development. it also shows how you nurture yourself.
(iii) the moon in astrology is the planet of emotion, senses, habits, intuition, security, and the inner child.

[5] (i) in the tarot deck, strength (reversed) represents that we have no power over our current situation. it can mean we have little personal strength or boundaries and refers to internal weaknesses we carry.
this card reminds us we can't control everything that happens in our lives, sometimes having to step back or withhold ourselves until a difficult, untamed period of life blows over.
(ii) the fifth house is an area of astrology which represents creative energy, the heart, pleasure, hobbies, drama, self-expression, attention, wildness, a lust for life, popularity and romance.
(iii) the sun in astrology is the planet of identity, ego, character, pride, vitality and individuality.

[6] (i) in the tarot deck, the hermit represents a period of withdrawal and detachment in order to find direction or truth in this world. this card suggests that introspection and solitude may be necessary before attempting to move forward in life. not necessarily a negative card, but it is essential to take this path when called upon so we can find the answers we need to grow.
(ii) the sixth house is an area of astrology which represents health, duties, structure, routines, purification, detail, and service to others.
(iii) mercury in astrology is the planet of communication, intelligence, skills, analysis, thought processes and logic.

[7] karmic debt nineteen: karmic numbers apply to birth dates but also can apply to the degrees on your birth chart placements e.g. virgo moon 19°. this karmic debt indicates that you may have mistreated others in your past life, through manipulation or the misuse of power. in order to pay off your debt in this life, you must help people, humble yourself to rely on others and apply your talent for hard work positively through acts of service. those who have karmic debt 19 have a tendency towards righteousness, narcissism, vanity and a strong desire for independence. this karma also reminds you that you are not an island, and that people can use help and support in healthy ways.

[8] (i) in the tarot deck, justice (reversed) represents a time in life where deeper meanings and the truth are being withheld by higher powers for reasons we cannot understand yet. logical, rational and just order may seem to be out of our grasp and we must wait for the truth to be revealed and justice to be granted.
(ii) the seventh house is an area of astrology which represents relationships, partnerships, alliances, contracts, bonds and how our interactions with others become part of our destiny.
(iii) venus in astrology is the planet of pleasure, love, relationships, values, beauty, affection, and our feminine energy.

[9] karmic debt sixteen: karmic numbers apply to birth dates but also can apply to the degrees on your birth chart placements e.g. libra rising 16°. this karmic debt indicates that you were egotistical in a past life and also had relationship issues where you struggled with intimacy and emotional connections. your karma in this life is to resolve your issues by becoming more thoughtful of others. any difficulties maintaining relationships may be because of issues with alienating yourself through self-absorption.

[10] (i) in the tarot deck, death represents a transformative period of life where an old cycle is ending to make way for a new one, elimination of the negativity or plagues that have been holding us back from evolving. some people will find this card difficult or an unnerving process in life, but it is inevitable.
(ii) the eighth house is an area of astrology which represents mystery, birth, sexuality, transformation, inheritance, investments, legacies, secrets, power, and taboos.
(iii) pluto in astrology is the planet of power, rebirth, obsessions, sexuality, darkness, death, upheaval and transcendence.

[11] (i) in the tarot deck, fortune represents the higher powers of chance, luck, the unknown, and destiny in life. neither a positive nor negative card, it symbolises the unpredictability of luck. it reminds us that even when we feel on the wrong side of luck, we still have a role to play in our fate, can take responsibility for our choices and can learn from our misfortunes.
(i) the ninth house is an area of astrology which represents expansion, inspiration, education, luck, philosophy, religion, spirituality and law.
(iii) jupiter in astrology is the planet of optimism, luck, abundance, purpose, faith, morals and opportunities.

[12] karmic debt fourteen: this karmic debt indicates that you abused personal freedom in a past life through extremist behaviour, addiction, overindulgence and lack of accountability. in this life, you may suffer a lack of self-control, responsibility and avoid commitment to yourself or others. in order to redeem your karma, you must develop discipline and find responsibilities that still grant you the flexibility you desire.

[13] (i) in the tarot deck, the devil represents a dark or sinful side of human nature, one that is tempted by materialism, obsessions, and a hunger for power. this mindset operates with cynicism and manipulation. this card can signify we are avoiding the truth, choosing ignorance or refusing to take responsibility four bad behaviour in life.
(ii) the tenth house is an area of astrology which represents structure, tradition, fame, honours, achievements, professional path, discipline, father figures, prestige, social status, and role in society.
(iii) saturn in astrology is the planet of discipline, reality, limitations, obstacles, restrictions, karma and ambition.

[14] (i) in the tarot deck, the fool represents an enthusiastic, naïve and adventurous persona who ventures into the world overly idealistic and ignorant of the potential hardships we may face. this card is neither positive nor negative, but warns us that not everything is at it seems and to not let others take advantage of our immaturity.
(ii) the eleventh house is an area of astrology which represents society, progression, ideas, the collective, originality, idealism, invention, the future and networking.
(iii) uranus in astrology is the planet of change, eccentricity, disruption, freedom, innovation and inspiration.

[15] (i) in the tarot the deck, the moon represents an unclear mind that is lost in worries, illusions, deception, subconscious fears, doubts and feelings. this card emphasises the difference between intuition and imagination, but also the vulnerability and insecurity associated with our unhealed shadow self.
(ii) the twelfth house is an area of astrology which represents dreams, emotions, hidden desires, self-destruction, sleep, surrenders, escapism, mysteries, hidden agendas and mental health issues.
(iii) neptune in astrology is the planet of imagination, illusion, idealism, mysticism, spirituality, and the subconscious world.

[16] karmic debt thirteen: karmic numbers apply to birth dates but also can apply to the degrees on your birth chart placements e.g. pisces venus 13°. this karmic debt indicates that in your past life you were self-defeatist, complacent and lazy. in this life, you may find that you experience more hurdles and frustrations than normal, having to work extra hard to achieve anything. may struggle to find your calling in life and feel talents are repressed and difficult to harness. in order to overcome this karma, you must remain resilient in efforts to not give up and practice self-control and organisation in order to follow through.

Printed in Great Britain
by Amazon

42721293R00118